MW01253274

ROAR
of LIONS

HOW I HEALED MY BREAST CANCER:
AN INSIGHT INTO SPIRITUALITY

NAZMINA LADHANI

BALBOA
PRESS

A DIVISION OF HAY HOUSE

Copyright © 2013 Nazmina Ladhani.

All rights reserved. No part of this book may be used or reproduced by
any means, graphic, electronic, or mechanical, including photocopying,
recording, taping or by any information storage retrieval system
without the written permission of the publisher except in the case
of brief quotations embodied in critical articles and reviews.

Balboa Press books may be ordered through booksellers or by contacting:

Balboa Press
A Division of Hay House
1663 Liberty Drive
Bloomington, IN 47403
www.balboapress.com
1-(877) 407-4847

Because of the dynamic nature of the Internet, any web addresses or
links contained in this book may have changed since publication and
may no longer be valid. The views expressed in this work are solely those
of the author and do not necessarily reflect the views of the publisher,
and the publisher hereby disclaims any responsibility for them.

The author of this book does not dispense medical advice or prescribe the use
of any technique as a form of treatment for physical, emotional, or medical
problems without the advice of a physician, either directly or indirectly. The
intent of the author is only to offer information of a general nature to help
you in your quest for emotional and spiritual well-being. In the event you use
any of the information in this book for yourself, which is your constitutional
right, the author and the publisher assume no responsibility for your actions.

Any people depicted in stock imagery provided by Thinkstock are models,
and such images are being used for illustrative purposes only.
Certain stock imagery © Thinkstock.

Printed in the United States of America

ISBN: 978-1-4525-6901-7 (sc)
ISBN: 978-1-4525-6900-0 (e)

Library of Congress Control Number: 2013903048

Balboa Press rev. date: 4/19/2013

I would like to dedicate this book to the loving memory of my mother, Fatmabai, my brother Jimmy (Abdul), and my nephew Rafiq Rajabali, who have all died of cancer.

I would like to thank Canadian author Susan Kingsbury, Azmina Jiwa, Fatima Thobani and Nicole Marois for inspiring and supporting me. And I would like to thank my special relatives Salim Jiwa, Micky Manji and Roshan Jiwa, as well as my friends, for being in my life.

Table of Contents

Preface

Any hurdle that comes in your life has to be considered a blessing, as it gives you an opportunity to change yourself. Change in life can affect you emotionally and culturally. There is a saying that change is good for you so you have to take complete charge of yourself. Change can also create lots of stress in one's life. We humans are so habit oriented that change can be difficult. It takes us away from our comfort zone. It takes us away from the things we are used to doing every day. Change can bring us into a different environment.

In order to adapt to change, one has to be in charge. One has to prepare mentally by thinking positive, as thoughts can be very powerful. But thinking positive is not easy, as it can be superficial while the negative continues to lie beneath the surface. In order to think positive, one has to release all the emotions from the body and get rid of all the past baggage that's been obscuring one's mind. In order to change, one has to work on oneself all the time. When change is done in a positive way, it can bring lots of new ideas and the mind can become more creative. The mind can be inspired by new things in life. This kind of feeling lifts up your spirits, and your body feels very good, which enhances your health.

It also makes you a stronger person. It gives you an opportunity to try to discover who you are and why this is happening to you. This way, you try to find out more about who you really are and why you have come to this earth. It gives a notion of spiritualism. It gets you more connected with the source and allows you to be on the spiritual path.

Introduction

The impact of the doctor's message was like *the roar of lions*. I was in shock, devastated, and scared. Breast cancer had never crossed my mind. My reaction to the news was the same reaction that you would have to the roar of lions in a jungle. You try to put the sound out of your mind, but you can't help but listen. The lions become your focus. The same was true for me with my cancer. I didn't want to be negative about it or focus on it, yet it became the focal point of my life over the next few years.

Initially, I had the same thoughts as many other women with cancer. I thought about dying or losing my hair, being away from work, the side effects of treatment, and the reaction of family and friends. How was I going to get through all of this? Over time, I developed survival techniques to help me through this difficult period. It is these techniques that I wish to share with you.

One of the biggest changes that I made in my life was to develop a stronger spiritual outlook and, in particular, to do more meditating. Practicing the various concentration and breathing techniques was a way for me to remain relaxed and connect with my creator. It was also a way for me to bring a positive focus to my life that enabled me to have hope for the future. I was no longer fearful of what was ahead of me. I was on a path toward inner peace and healing.

But I also used other techniques, such as eating well and exercising more. I tried to take a more holistic approach to my life and made changes that would ultimately improve my daily well-being and long-term health. Exercise included everything from long walks to swimming, light yoga for stretching and toning. And after each session, I felt better and stronger. I could feel my body, spirit, and mind working together to make me well fighting the cancer.

Having breast cancer has been a journey for me. After nine years of health, I know now, more than ever before, that I can meet any challenge that comes my way. I'm strong mentally, spiritually, and physically. I continue with all the good habits that I formed during my illness, and I continue to benefit from them.

The purpose of this book is to share with you the techniques that I have learned on my journey. I hope that they can also help you in such a way that the "roar of lions" will disappear in your life. And I wish you as much success with your journey as I have had on mine.

Chapter 1

Personal Story: Entering the Jungle

Have you ever had a perfect morning? One where the sun was shining brightly, the sky was clear and blue, and the air was fresh? I had such a day. It was a stunningly beautiful Saturday morning with a clear, azure sky—an absolutely perfect summer's day. At that time, I had already been off work due to another health issue and was in Toronto for a "recuperation" weekend. I had activities planned and was looking forward to a fun and relaxing time. Little did I know then that my life was about to change.

While taking a refreshing shower on that superb summer morning, I discovered three lumps in a cluster in my right breast on the side leading toward the armpit.

The cluster wasn't visible with the naked eye (I had checked in the mirror), but I could certainly feel them when I touched the area. I was understandably surprised, but at the same time, I was not overly alarmed. I knew that many lumps are benign, and certainly, I wasn't going to worry about them at this point. I didn't even know how long the cluster had been there, as I had not been doing regular checkups on myself. Of course, this was the first lesson I learned—always do regular checkups. Deciding not to pay too much attention to it at that moment, I was determined to be as positive as possible. Lots of fun things had been planned for this weekend and I'd really been looking forward to it for a long time, so nothing was going to spoil it.

The first step when I returned to Ottawa was to consult with my family doctor. His initial impression was that they looked benign, but to be on the safe side, he recommended tests at the hospital. The appointment was two weeks away.

During those two weeks, I decided that the best medicine for me was to take control of this issue and the first step on my journey was to remain positive. I worked hard at trying to train my self-conscious to work with my body in sending and receiving positive messages. I continually told myself that the lumps were not cancerous. This had put me more in a better frame of mind for my appointment.

My goal right from the start was always to be as healthy as I could be. I have always felt that worrying is a waste of energy. I needed my body and mind to work together on this issue, so it was important to be positive no matter what came my way. I wanted to have a good perspective, be able to see things clearly, and remain calm, so that I would be better able to make the right decisions along the way. Especially if the news was that I had cancer. It was going to be mind over matter.

When I went for my mammogram, I was mentally ready. I wanted the test so that we could determine my state of health. The test went well, but the results still were not very clear. I was a bit apprehensive, but I always believe that worrying is a waste of energy. I controlled myself and trusted enough in me to look ahead in a positive manner.

The next step was to have a biopsy so that a more accurate reading could be made. I had to wait almost a week for my results. The waiting wasn't very pleasant, but I relied on positive thinking to get me through. Again, I wanted to be in the best frame of mind to receive my results.

> "Healing is a matter of time, but it is sometimes also a matter of opportunity."

> Hippocrates

CHAPTER 2

Diagnosis: Roar of the Lions

I was at work feeling a bit apprehensive, as my mind was wandering. A week had passed by since my biopsy, and somehow I felt that my results must be in at the doctor's office. I had an intuition that something was wrong. In the midafternoon, I called the doctor's office and was told they would call me back. This raised a big question mark.

Finally, the big moment arrived. The doctor phoned me and said that the results of the biopsy were positive: I had breast cancer. The next step was to see the oncologist in nine days. The doctor also said that surgery would be performed, but he couldn't tell me what kind. I had to go and see the doctor.

It was around 4:30 p.m. and I was at work. My first reaction was to talk to my supervisor. She was affable and very sympathetic and offered me to drive to the doctor, but I did not accept the offer. I thought I could handle it on my own.

I left work and walked toward my car, where I felt guided to check my tires. I was amazed to see one tire was almost flat. Luckily, there was a gas station with a garage next to the parking lot. I drove my car to the garage and the problem was fixed after removing the glass from the tire; the mechanic was able to patch the tire. It was around 6:00 p.m., so I decided to phone the doctor and explained the situation. After talking with the doctor, I felt it was a blessing in disguise. Otherwise, I could have gotten stuck in traffic. But the obstacle of the tire facilitated me going straight home.

I was shocked and devastated, and for the first time, I could hear the roar of the lions. My reaction to the news was the same as if I had heard the roar of lions in a jungle. I would try to ignore the roaring, but I would likely still listen. The lions would become my focus. I was mentally prepared, but at the same time, it certainly wasn't a message that I wanted to hear. I couldn't help feeling a sense of uncertainty, and I was worried about such things as losing my hair, being off work, the side effects from treatment, the reaction of family and friends, and the possibility of death. I simply couldn't believe that it was happening to me. I felt that my brain and my thoughts were out of control. Yet I knew that I had to silence the lions as much as possible and remain hopeful.

I talked with other women who had gone through cancer. They were feeling sorry for me, not being encouraging or constructive. Their stories just made me feel worse and even more discouraged. I felt timid and had lost my self-confidence. Although I knew that somebody else's experience, good or bad, does not necessarily apply to me, their stories still influenced my emotions.

I am a strong believer that one who feels sorry for oneself has no control over oneself, so I had to be in control. Instead of being entangled in this situation, I had to step back. I had to see what my perspective was. By being detached, I could see the perspective. By stepping back and seeing the situation, I felt more in control and in charge. By going back again in the situation, I was more in control with my emotions. With meditation and breathing, I felt even more in charge.

Additionally, at that moment, I did not know if the cancer had spread or not. This was another worry and another thing that I had to prepare for. During the night, I was flooded with negative thoughts to the point that I did not have a peaceful sleep.

During those two weeks, the roar of lions was encircling me, but I had to go back to basics, which for me was to think positive. It was my primary survival technique. Positive thinking is easy to do when life is going well and you are happy. But the test is when you are faced with a major life challenge. Knowing the implications from having breast cancer conjures up many negative feelings, so it is hard to think positively during those times. Yet I knew in my heart that unless I did something fundamental to relax my body, I would continue to feel depressed and negative and make the situation worse. In the end, it was up to me to take control, and that is what I did.

The next day, I went to work with an optimistic outlook so that I wouldn't burden anybody with my problem. For the most part, I kept to myself. However, I took advantage of the beautiful sunny day and decided to go for lunch with my coworker. I found it soothing to sit beside the river while I ate a healthy salad. I told my friend I had breast cancer, and she was shocked to see how well I was handling it. I felt that her comments confirmed that my breathing exercises were working. If I was being positive on the inside, it should therefore show on the outside in my appearance. I felt I was on the right path to health.

That evening, I had an appointment with my chiropractor and talked to him about my cancer. That was the best thing I did, because he was very supportive of my situation and gave me a book on how to fight cancer with nutrition. Every evening, I read that book and it helped me, giving me the strength to fight the cancer. I followed a vegetarian diet instantly. I hung in there for nine days, doing my breathing exercises, which gave me lots of energy. For me, the goal was to focus on getting well. Negative thoughts would have only drained me completely, which would, of course, make the disease worse.

The big day finally came for me to see the oncologist. In a way, I felt that I had been waiting forever. That morning, I woke up early feeling a bit nervous. I took a shower, had breakfast, and left at eight o'clock in order to make it for my appointment at nine o'clock. I was surprised to see the heavy traffic on the bridge. It was September and the colors of the trees were changing, so it looked immaculate around the Ottawa River. I have an affinity for water and everything around started to look attractive. The sky was clear, and a clear sky in the morning was an auspicious sign on the day of my appointment.

Surprisingly enough, I panicked, thinking that I wouldn't make my appointment. If I missed it, then I would have to wait longer to see him. At this point, my intuition kicked in. It directed me to take the second lane, which is designated for a taxi or two people in a car. I took that lane, and by chance, there was no sign of police that morning. Luckily, I made it for my appointment on time.

CHAPTER 3

Treatment: Entering the Lion's Den

The cancer specialist was a young man from London, England. He was a very professional and friendly doctor, and we had a good personality match right from the beginning. Given that the appointment was at a teaching hospital, he also had an assistant student doctor with him and was explaining everything to her at the same time.

At the round table in his office, he shared the results of my test with me. He explained these by giving me an example of a slope ending in the river. He explained that at the present moment, we were at the top of the hill and we did not know what the condition of the water was down at the bottom of the hill, as it was obscure, unclear,

11

and clouded. He had a very philosophical explanation, which made a lot of sense. Only during the operation, when he removed the lump, would he know more, such as whether the cancer had spread, how far, and whether I would need a mastectomy or not. As it happened, there was a cancellation, so my operation was scheduled for two days later. So luckily, I did not have to wait long; otherwise, the encircling of the lion would be elusive.

Before leaving the hospital, I was asked by the head nurse if I had any issues, and my main issue was taking time off from work as I only had two weeks of sick leave left. I was in this room where this nice nurse was and was planning to discuss my future concerning time off from work and my finances. I felt claustrophobic and excused myself from the room. I just wanted to go home to my cozy nest.

After I left the hospital, I was very emotional and cried; I was very worried. Before I left the hospital, I was given a book about cancer-stricken people who had gone through the operation with different scenarios.

After reading this book at night, I was becoming weak and depressed. I was thinking of the worst happening to me, as some of the pictures were not pleasant—the pictures where mastectomies had been performed. Also, the stories of couples—how their lives changed after having cancer and they managed to cope with it. It took them a few years to have normal lives again. Some of them had to go to counseling in order to live a normal life again. In order for me not to hear the lions, I listened to the audio tape *Cancer: Discover Your Healing Power,* by Louise Hay, which helped me tremendously.

The following day, instead of being dismal, I took it easy and meditated. I did yoga, which was comprised of different breathing techniques, stretching, and toning of my body. I listened to the tapes of Louise Hay, which inspired me to prepare a nice dinner and be healthful. I pampered myself by taking a tub bath with a gentle aroma in the air and lit candles around the tub; I felt pleasantly calm and peaceful. I felt blessed to have the feeling of pleasantness. I felt ready for my operation the next morning.

Chapter 4

Facing the Lions

When I woke up in the morning, I could still hear the birds of September. I felt peaceful and connected with nature.

My operation was at 8:00 a.m., and afterward, the doctor said it was successful. He said that it did not seem like the cancer had spread, but my biopsy still had to be tested, and I would have my results in a week.

Out of the three lumps, only one was cancerous. At that moment, I counted my blessings. I felt content and blessed to have this oncologist as my surgeon. Also, I was blessed to have my friends who came to visit me and showered me with flowers and goodies. Well, I said,

"What more can I ask?" I was alone in Ottawa, yet I never felt alone.

My seven lymph nodes were removed and sent for testing at the laboratory. At home, I tried to heal myself, and I had to do the exercises for my arm by moving my fingers against the wall, climbing up and down, which would help my pectoral muscles. I did this religiously in order not to have any defects with my arm. In the beginning, it was very hard, as my arm could not go all the way up on the wall because the lymph nodes under my arms had been removed. I was not being sluggish when it came to exercising my arm, but I was genial. My operation did not stop me from taking daily showers, which slowly removed the patch that was on the stitches where my lump had been removed. In other words, I had a lumpectomy and my stitches started to dissolve.

With sheer determination, it started healing. I was feeling positive again because of my breathing exercises. I was the fan of my own club. My tenacious effort in meditating and doing yoga helped me to tap into the field of pure potentiality and practice silence, which helped my healing process. It also made me feel supported by the universe, which helped me a lot. It made me cope with the lions.

After a bit more than a week, I had an appointment with the oncologist again, and I was showered with the good news that I was healing well and my lymph nodes had tested negative. This was a huge relief for me, and I thanked God for it. I have always believed in the saying that "God helps those who help themselves." I was told that I would be contacted by the other oncologists, who would talk to me about chemotherapy and radiation therapy.

I had an appointment with the chemo oncologist. I had a discussion with her regarding what would happen if I did not take the chemo. I was a little dubious about chemo in the beginning but decided it was my best option after the consultation with my chemo oncologist.

In the beginning, I decided to take a slow chemo and was given some oral chemo tablets that I took for a week. On the third day, which was Wednesday, I was feeling terrible. I had called the hospital about my feelings and they said that it was normal. By Saturday, I was feeling terrible and talked to one doctor who said it was normal. I had an intuition that something was wrong, but I did not follow my intuition. I deviated from the spiritual path. I could have done some research on the tablets, including the side effects and relation to the bone marrow, in order to find out why was I feeling so awful.

It was a dark moment in my journey. I felt I was going to die.

Finally, after a week I had an appointment with the chemo oncologist. From the blood test, it was discovered that my bone marrow was sensitive to chemo and had stopped producing new white cells. I was asked to immediately stop taking the chemo tablets. The chemo oncologist wished I had not taken the tablets that morning. During that week, I really suffered due to my white cells being destroyed and not reproducing.

In order to have chemo, I was told I would have to have injections, which would produce the white cells, and then medical professionals would give me the chemo, which would kill the white cells. I was ambivalent about having chemo. I felt like just a number, as if chemo was given to every cancer patient. I am very glad that, in the end, I decided not to take chemotherapy. But the chemo oncologist was not very happy with my decision and said sarcastically that I never wanted to take chemo from the beginning.

Even after the chemo oncologist's negative remarks, I still felt positive about my decision: my lymph nodes had tested negative and my cancer had not spread. I decided to take radiation therapy only, which made so much sense to me, as it would kill any cancer cells that were left after the surgery. I was scheduled for radiation therapy three months after my surgery, starting on January 15. I would get it every day for four weeks, excluding weekends.

Two months after my surgery in September, my brother Jimmy (Abdul) died in London, England, of lung cancer. I flew to London for the funeral.

It was strange to be at his funeral. Here he had died from cancer, and I was hopefully on the road to recovery. Interestingly, if I had still been on chemo, I would have been too ill to travel. I was lucky to have been there. I met the family and my aunt who I had not seen for years. Her jovial nature helped to lighten the situation. Participating in all the funeral ceremonies gave me lots of internal peace.

My brother was a kind soul. He took life very easy, smoked all his life, and his reaction to cancer was not frightful. In his case, the cancer was very aggressive and therefore spread very fast; he probably did not have much time to think about it. He is in a better place now.

My radiation therapy was only going to start in January. So a few days after my brother's funeral, I went to Phaphos on Cyprus, an island on the Mediterranean, for a week. My room was on the ground floor right in front of the Mediterranean.

In the evening when I arrived, it was raining and the scenery looked spectacular, with palm trees swirling around the sea and the warm breeze caressing my cheeks. I felt naturally peaceful.

While in Phaphos, I woke up in the morning and took a stroll on the Mediterranean, which connected me to nature, and I felt so connected to nature that I felt I was nourishing nature and nature was nourishing me. After a stroll, I had breakfast, and it was a week of rejuvenation: lying on the deck in front of the sea and listening to the healing tapes, which helped me a lot and put me in a positive mood.

Since I love swimming, I took advantage of the facilities and swam for two hours every afternoon before English tea and biscuits were served at four o'clock in the hotel lobby. I was surrounded by cheerful people, mainly from London, England. My mind was clear, and I felt everyone was so wonderful. I felt I was on a spiritual journey. I feel this whole trip really helped me to relax, and of course, this must have boosted my immune system.

When I came back in January, my body eagerly responded to the treatment. I felt my body start to heal itself. I took my radiation therapy for four weeks. I started drinking warm milk with turmeric powder before the radiation therapy and continued to do so during the treatment, which is beneficial to the body. Turmeric powder is explained in tip number 1.

Along the way, there were a number of bumps, but at least I got through them. One unpleasant outcome was the burn I had to deal with from radiation therapy.

I had a burn at the bottom of my breast, which happened just before the last treatment. It was not as bad as some I had heard about. In many cases, the burn starts to appear midway through the treatment. However, the best part was the burn didn't hurt. I should say that the burn appeared only toward the end of the treatment. The burn could not heal while the treatment was still going on, as it just got worse. After my treatment, it took almost a week for the burn to heal. No scar is left because I used the oil from vitamin E tablets. I do not call this being lucky or happening by chance, because I controlled my emotions and have always believed that every cloud has a silver lining.

CHAPTER 5

Recovery

The good news is that I have been cancer free for nine years. I feel good and am looking forward to the future. After nine years, I can say that this has been quite the journey. I have learned a lot of life lessons along the way and have met many kind people. Often I had dark moments, but they didn't stay. I worked hard at having an optimistic outlook, and it paid off. I forced out the roar of lions and tamed them. And now I am stronger than ever and ready to take on the world.

CHAPTER 6

Things to Know (Lymphatic System)

When I was diagnosed with breast cancer, I was told I would have an operation to remove the lump and my lymph nodes would be removed. Lymph nodes would be tested in the laboratory to find out if the cancer had spread or not, but at that time, I did not know what the function of the lymph nodes was.

The research I did was on breast cancer, chemo, and radiation, what the latter two do, and their side effects. But I never studied lymph nodes.

CHAPTER 7

Lymph Nodes

Often, breast cancer patients also have to deal with complications after cancer, if the lumph nodes have been removed. One of them is a blockage in the lymphatic system, a condition called lymphedema. Most people do not know what lymphedema is until they have it. Once diagnosed, they are shocked and concerned about what to do.

I had such a blockage. To my surprise, I had never heard about lymphedema. After looking at Internet pictures of people who had lymphedema, I felt timid. Having this complication gave me another challenge to face while fighting breast cancer. Again, I tried to keep the "roar of lions" at bay.

There are several different options for the treatment of lymphedema, including various kinds of compression garments. Doctors often recommend them to prevent swelling.

Simply put, the lymphatic system consists of lymph nodes that act as filters to clean our blood. Usually, the fluid travels upward in the body and passes through the lymph nodes that clean it, and then it goes to the heart

This sounds like a simple process, but when something goes wrong with this flow, health problems occur. As I said earlier, I had a one-inch cancerous lump that was at the second level. Doctors performed a lumpectomy, which means that they removed my lump and seven lymph nodes. And I had radiation therapy. In so doing, some scar tissue remained under my arm. Radiation enhanced tightness around my under arm where the lymph nodes had been removed. These changes resulted in a lot of tightness around that area, to the point that it was blocking the flow of fluid. Therefore, fluid was not passing through for cleaning. And to make matters worse, gravity played a role, as it was pulling the fluid down to my hand. Hence, my arm swelled.

At that point, I realized that I had to take action. It wasn't going to heal itself on its own. Luckily, after a few phone calls, I found a rehabilitation center with experts in this field. This center played a key role in my road to recovery.

The first step was to have a consultation with a therapist, which took one hour. With such a thorough consultation, I had confidence in what they could do for me. After the consultation, the therapist explained the cause of the blockage and then told me that mine was reversible.

In terms of blockage, the therapists use a scale, and lucky for me, my level was only from zero to one. Up to level one, they can reverse it by creating new channels, but if it has reached level two or three, it's not reversible. And other complications can emerge. At that point, you live with it your whole life and need ongoing lymphatic massages and treatment for lymphedema, including various kinds of compression garments. One of these is a "sleeve" that one wears on the arm. It looks more like a stocking with natural colors to match the skin. Doctors recommend it to prevent swelling.

So what does creating new channels mean? Let me begin with an analogy of a stream of water. When there is a stream of water in the woods and something is put in it to block the flow of water, usually the stream will begin to create other routes so the water keeps flowing. New streams develop. This same approach is applied to the lymphatic fluid by creating new channels; the lymphatic massage is routed toward new channels until they are built and the flow is steady. Also, lymphatic massage causes the tightness and the scar tissue to go away, which also helps the flow of the lymphatic fluid.

After working with the therapist for three months, she was able to get the fluid to move on its own. This procedure took some time, given that the area had scar tissue and was swelling. In the beginning, my appointments took place three times a week, but they started to decrease as we began to see results. One important thing that I learned was that if I had gone to the therapist after my radiation treatment, there would have been less chance of my arm swelling. Doctors would have controlled it early in my treatment.

At the moment, my lymphatic fluid is moving on its own. But stress and negative thoughts can slow the flow of the fluid so that I would be able to feel it right away. Amazingly, my hand is doing so well now due to my yoga poses, which are comprised of half-moon and warrior poses that open up the shoulders and loosen the tightness around it.

I am so convinced that meditation and yoga have enhanced my healing process.

CHAPTER 8

How to Take Care of Yourself

The physician takes care of the curing process. This includes various methods, such as surgery and giving pills. On the other hand, healing is spiritual, which involves one's thoughts, behavior, attitude, and lots of different methods that I have explained in the tips below.

"God helps those who help themselves."

Ben Franklin

CHAPTER 9

Taming the Lions: Tips

The purpose of this chapter is to provide you with some tips that I found helpful along my journey, and I still use many of them today. Each tip helped me quiet the roar of lions and led me on a path of wellness while building up my immune system.

> "We are not human beings having a
> spiritual experience; we are spiritual
> beings having a human experience."

Telhard de Chardin, a french philosopher

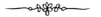

Tip No. 1
Turmeric Powder

"Success doesn't come to you; you must go to it."

Marva Collins

Before my radiation therapy, I prepared myself by eating good food—lots of vegetables—and drinking milk with an Indian spice—turmeric—every night. I warmed the milk and added a quarter teaspoon of turmeric powder.

> "Turmeric is a very powerful healer. It's an ingredient in curry powder, which Asians have used for a long time as a stomach tonic, a blood purifier, a skin treatment, and for healing wounds. Today it is potentially beneficial in treating or reducing symptoms associated with a wide range of health conditions. It has antioxidant, antitumor, anti-inflammatory, and antibacterial effects."[1]

---

1   How Is Turmeric Used in Ayurvedic Medicine?" Joan Firstenberg. Demand Media, Inc. Accessed on 13 December, 2012.

Tip No. 2
Yoga

I have done my yoga training at Chopra Center, Carlsbad, California. I am a qualified yoga teacher. Yoga has really helped me in my healing process. Yoga is union of mind, body, and soul, or spirituality. To put it into perspective about mind, body, and soul, physical and emotional baggage creates toxicity and does not help a disease like cancer. With the personal experience, I can say that the other name of yoga is healing. It intoxicates you when your mind, body, and soul are unionized. It gives a feeling of complete blankness, and you can feel the body is healing.

> "Spiritual practices connect us to our unbounded selves, and in so doing, elicit a deep relaxation response in our mindbody. When we are in a state of deep relaxation and connection, our entire physiology has the potential to change.
>
> A study published in 2008 by researchers at Massachusetts General Hospital and Harvard Medical School was the first to document the fact that practices of meditation and yoga can

affect gene expression. The researchers were able to show that by engaging in spiritual practices, we can turn on (express) healthy genes and turn off (not express) harmful genes. The study found that the practice of meditation, yoga, deep breathing, and prayer can change the expression of thousands of genes. The genes that are affected are those that control inflammation and cell death, as well as those involved in how the body deals with abnormal cells".[2]

Yoga is all about breathing and stretching. I have learned different kinds of breathing, namely *ujay* breathing, *bastrika* breathing, *clear* breathing, five-pointed star breathing, *kundilini* breathing, and so forth. All of these different kinds of breathing help the lungs, stomach, and heart to become stronger. They also help one to achieve self-awareness. When mind, body, and soul come together, one awakens to the higher state of consciousness.

2   Sheila Patel, M.D. and Valencia Porter, M.D., M.P.H., "Mind-Body Approaches to Preventing Breast Cancer" *Chopra Centre Newsletter*, October 2012.

Different *asanas* (poses) enhance muscle flexibility. With each asana, breathe in and stay for a few seconds in the pose. The breath can help one to go deeper into the pose. While stretching into the pose and breathing consciously, oxygen helps the whole body become flexible. With practice, the spine becomes flexible, which is the fountain of youth.

Chakras are the energy centers, the meridian from the head to the base of the spine. Chakras are associated with rainbow colors: red, orange, yellow, green, blue, indigo, and violet. There are seven chakras. Each chakra is associated with a sound and color. The following are the seven chakras one needs to awaken by the concept of breathing in and paying attention to the relevant chakra, as well as saying the sound associated with that particular chakra. For example, one says, *"Lammm."* Where our attention goes, energy flows, awakening each chakra.

- At the base of the spine, the root chakra, when it is awakened, gives us a feeling of being more grounded and stable in life, which is red in color. The sound is *lam*.

- Below the belly button, which is a creative and a sexual chakra, this is orange in color. The sound is *vam*.

- Above the belly button, below the heart, which is a solar plexus chakra giving a lot of energy, self-esteem, etc. This is bright yellow in color, and the sound is *ram*.

- Heart chakra, when awakened, gives harmony, compassion, and love so that it can flow back and forth easily. This is green in color, and the sound is *yum*.

- Throat chakra, when awakened, helps the thyroid glands and improves the communication skill. This is blue in color, and the sound is *hum*.

- Between the eyes, the third eye, which is an intuition chakra, improves insights and develops our psychic ability. This is violet in color, and the sound is *sham*.

- Infinite chakra, on top of the crown, is the ability to fully connect spiritually, which is violet in color. The sound is *ohm,* which is a universal and does not have any meaning.

When these energy centers are blocked, energy cannot flow freely, which means that disease can appear. It is important to tone the chakras with different sounds related to different chakras.

Tip No. 3
Living a Spiritual Life

Spirituality is a favorable or promising sign of healing. In order to heal, one should have an attitude of love, inclusiveness, and harmony. It is about knowing who you really are. It is about acceptance and accepting what transpires in life and being the person you should be. Also, it is about accepting the rhythm of life by embracing it and finding the opportunities within.

According to me, to be on a spiritual path is not to carry any ego. It is to be forgiving and loving. It is to focus on the positivity that life offers and to face the challenges with courage.

When one is on a spiritual path, one is less sensitive to the issues in life and also more accommodating and accepting of people as they are. Being spiritual helps the healing process by promoting positive energy. Being despondent, apprehensive, or fearful harms the body.

Spirituality comes from within. I have always known this and had to work hard to be my own "fan" club. I couldn't rely on other people to generate my spirituality. It is important not to have high expectations from other people when you are going through your cancer. This way, you will feel less disappointed. But more importantly, you will keep in control of your life.

Tip No. 4
Learn to Breathe Properly

Breathing properly has both physical and psychological benefits. It takes the stomach and the nose to work as a team and in harmony. The stomach acts as the energy source while the nose acts like a natural filtrating system. First, take a deep breath through your nose, mouth closed, and at the same time inflate your stomach. Second, hold your breath for a few seconds. Third, as you exhale slowly, press your belly button toward your spine such that you contract your stomach. This process helps to move energy throughout your body, which ultimately rejuvenates your muscles and tissues. Additionally, this breathing technique can be used as a form of meditation or simply as a way to calm the mind. With practice, it will come automatically and you will enjoy the benefits.

I am following a degree course at University of Metaphysical Sciences in California. The following is the extract from University of Metaphysical Sciences

"There are three types of breathing, which I will explain more as we move farther into this material: thoracic breathing (mid chest), clavicular breathing (upper chest), and diaphragmatic breathing (belly, abdomen).

Thoracic breathing (chest breathing) fills only the middle and upper portion of the lungs and not the lower portions, where most of the blood is. Clavicular Breathing is centered around the collarbones and only comes into play when the body needs great amounts of oxygen, for instance, while exercising.

Diaphragmatic breathing is the most efficient breathing there is. This is because most of the blood is circulating in the lower parts of the lung and oxygen infusion is mostly happening there. The diaphragmatic breathing pulls the oxygen lower into the lungs, increasing the efficiency of oxygen infusion into the blood stream because the oxygen is exposed to more of the blood. Interestingly, children and infants do this naturally. It is only later that adult humans stop using this most efficient way of breathing."[3]

To maximize my healing, I practice my breathing exercise as long as I am comfortable and add gentle, pleasant, natural fragrance to the environment, which adds to my relaxation. Pay attention to your breathing and invite the body and mind by allowing the oxygen to travel to different areas of your body. First let it flow to your head, neck, and shoulders, and then down your arms to the tips of your fingers and back, and finally to your pelvis and down your legs to the tips of your toes.

Once you feel relaxed and are in a good frame of mind, focus on your breathing. Say to yourself that you are feeling good about yourself, and visualize the roar of lions that is slowly going away. Continue breathing and

3   Breese, Christian D.D., Ph.D., "Pranayama & The Art of Breathing" University of Metaphysical Sciences, 2005

say to yourself that you are the best, you love yourself, you have lots of potential and courage, and you have let go of all resentment, jealousy, or evil. Feel free. Be calm, be silent, and be receptive to other signs that you are part of a universe.

Every breath in your body will release any tension from your body. Stretch your body and it will be flexible. The roar of lions is slowly disappearing, and you do not hear it anymore. You will feel wonderful and reborn. It is important to do this breathing regimen every day to heal yourself. But just as importantly, this technique is a lifetime commitment that will enhance your well-being.

The good news is that the healing process can continue all your life, whether you are cancer free or not, and you can do it anywhere and anytime. To get started, play your favorite music, sit in a comfortable position, close your eyes, and take in a deep breath. Feel your body begin to relax. Tell your consciousness to let go of any resentment that you have in your life and any fear that you have. These can be like dark clouds hanging over you and can take away the positive energy from your body. Try to feel the rhythm of the universe. Be still, listen, and breathe. According to research, new cells develop in our bodies every few weeks; through the breathing and positive energy, new healthy cells can replace cancer cells. By listening to the inspirational tapes, I learned that one cancer patient had used breathing and positive thinking to remove cancer by herself. Cancer cells do not prefer oxygenated tissues. Cancer cells are abnormal cells that can develop from stress and the daily hustle and bustle of life.

Tip No. 5
Thoughts Can Be Very Powerful

The thought manifest as the word;
The word manifests as the deed;
The deed develops into habit;
And habit hardens into character.
So watch the thought and its way with care.
And let it spring from love
Born out of concern for all beings.

Buddha

If thoughts are related to arguments, this can affect the breathing, as mind and body are connected. Any negative thoughts will result in disrupted breathing, which can affect the health of the body. Happy thoughts will improve the breathing, which rejuvenates the cells.

Thoughts can be very powerful; whatever you think can transfer into reality. To put it into perspective, be more open toward your thinking. My thoughts were very simple and made my healing easier. As thoughts can be very powerful, any ill thoughts can be portrayed very easily without paying much attention to them. For example, ill thoughts are talking negative and being critical about others. I was aware that while the brain processed thoughts, visualization was taking place. At the same time, I thought and visualized my dreams, which were transpiring into reality, and the lions were disappearing from my thoughts.

I always believe that negative thinking results in greater negativity, whereas positive thinking improves health, prospects, creativity, and more. With the ill thoughts, the frame of the mind changes and the tone of the voice changes. And it can come out in a rude manner portrayed in an angry form unknowingly.

Anger is negative and a sign of insecurity. But when you are thinking positive, you are feeling good, which changes your physiology. And in turn, your voice becomes low and pleasant. Any criticism or feedback can be absorbed in a very positive manner. A good frame of mind perceives life in a positive way. In order to enhance the good frame of mind, avoid being caught up in gossip or any ill thoughts about anything in life.

In my healing process, I couldn't think about the cancer. The thought of cancer in itself is a problem. Any thought put toward the unnecessary issues becomes a problem. So a problem can be created by us, and by attaching too much importance, it increases the stress in our body. Our mind and body can be inflamed, which enhances the abnormal cells (i.e., cancer cells). So let it be. Detach yourself from the problem, and continue doing deep breathing exercise. And in my case, it was disappearing by itself and I did not hear the roar of the lions in my ears.

Tip No. 6
Forgiveness

"People have to forgive. We don't have to like them, we don't have to be friends with them, we don't have to send them hearts in text messages, but we have to forgive them, to overlook, to forget. Because if we don't we are tying rocks to our feet, too much for our wings to carry!"

C. JoyBell C.

⌒⊶⟐⊶⌒

Forgiving and loving are the most cheerful and pleasant things to do. When someone has hurt you in any way, you have to forgive that person, as that person was probably not in his right mind regarding his actions. Or maybe that was the only way that person knew how to behave in that particular moment. Again, one should not be offended but be forgiving to others. Again we do have choices (whereas animals do not). One can say very confidently, "I am not going to get hurt if anybody says anything, as I have a choice not to get hurt and forgive that person." By practicing this, l felt great about myself.

At the end of the day, we are looking for peace in life, and this is one way of getting it.

Resentment is another type of disease. It is important to forgive, eliminate any resentment, and live in the present. Removing resentment from the body will enhance the healing process. The present moment is important, and once that moment is gone, do not look into that moment that has passed.

Forgiveness is another quality which can remove low energy from the body. This can help in the healing process. It also keeps your mind clear of the lions roaring.

Tip No. 7
Laughing

Laughter really is the best medicine! Norman Cousins, the famous author, found out that he had terminal cancer. Cousins did not want to hear the word *cancer* and started doing research. He found that the best remedy to cure cancer was good humor. So he surrounded himself with humor books, jokes books, and witty friends, and then he did lot of belly laughing. Laughter boosts the level of endorphins, the body's natural painkiller, and suppresses the stress hormone. The cancer did not stand a chance against all the good endorphins produced by the body. He came out of the hospital as a healthier man, and his cancer had disappeared.

There is a saying that "Laughter is the best medicine," and it is so true. Laughing and being happy form one of the best healing methods. Physiological studies also show that laughter increases the production of the body's own painkillers while at the same time increasing the immune system. It is good that happy family members and good friends who make us laugh surround us. Laughing enhances the release of the endorphins from the brain, relaxes the body and mind, and inspires us. It promotes the notion of living "in the present." Living in present puts us in a creative mode and will allow us to think of the present moment and how to improve it. We won't about the past and the future.

Most of the programs I watch on TV are comedy shows.

Tip No. 8
Kindness

"Be the living expression of … kindness, kindness
in your face, kindness in your eyes, kindness in
your smile, kindness in your warm greeting."

Mother Teresa of Calcutta

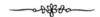

One way is being kind to all the creatures in the universe. Kindness is one of the greatest qualities one can possess.

I will give you an example of showing kindness. I had attended an inspirational seminar a few years back. The tickets were quite expensive. During this seminar, a lady was called on the stage and asked how she managed to come to this seminar. She said that she was three years cancer free and one of her friends, who was a waiter, had sent her three hundred dollars to spend it anyway she liked. She decided to attend this seminar. The speaker gave her a gift of one hundred fifty dollars toward the ticket. By showing this act of kindness to the lady, she felt very good and the people who witnessed this act of kindness felt good about themselves.

When one is feeling good about oneself, according to research, the brain releases a chemical called serotonin. Serotonin gives a very calming effect, and one feels better about oneself. By showing kindness, both parties benefit.

Tip No. 9
Detoxification

Detoxification of the body can also help in healing the body. I have a recipe for a soup that helps detoxification.

Detoxification Diet Vegetable Broth. Helps mineralize and alkalinize body

Boil 2 litres of water

Add 1 cup each of carrots, potatoes, parsely, kale, spinach, zucchini, Green beans, beetroot

Boil for 10-30 minutes

Remove the boiled vegetables and sip on half or 1 litre of soup daily

Eat vegetables separately

Use organic ingredients as much as possible.[4]

---

4   www.sunrisewellnesscentre.com 2004

CHAPTER 10

Added Tips

"Meditation calms our mind and makes it easier for us to pay attention to the reality around and within us."

Blaise Pascal

M editation is a practice that benefits mind, body, and spirit. Meditation requires discipline. When you are disciplined, meditation comes automatically. To put it into perspective, there is a relationship between soul and meditation. Meditation is food for the soul. When one feeds the soul regularly, one will always remain happy. When one does not feed the soul regularly, it somehow feels dissatisfied. The soul feels like a stranger in the body. It's the same as if you went to a big city and did not know anybody so you felt all alone. When you do not feed the soul properly, you feel unhappy too.

> "In order to meditate, concentrate on your breathing through the navel (stomach) and you have to be in the present moment. Try to focus between your two eyes. While breathing, *pingala* (surya) flows through the right nostril. *Ida* (chandra) flows through the left nostril. Both crisscross back and forth across the spine. *Sushumna* is the central pathway moving straight down the middle of the spine and is the moment when both nostrils are open and operating equally. When the breath arises from (in the state of enlightenment) the region of the navel inside the body, perform rhythmic inhaling and exhaling of air, which leads to spiritual joy and salvation. The meditative expansion of that moment is *sandhya*, a state in which sounds, thoughts, and other disturbances from within and without do not disturb the meditator.

It is a "magic moment" or "magic zone" at the base of the spine, in the root chakra, or *mudladhara*."[5]

While breathing, you can say any of the names of God. You can repeat this name with concentration. The repetition of the same sound eventually brings you into the gap.

Meditating can connect you with your soul. To know your soul is to know your higher self. By regularly meditating, you will ask, "Who am I and what is my purpose in life?" Do not try to find an answer through the mind. Keep looking inside yourself and asking the same question; your awareness will increase. Do not pay attention to the millions of thoughts that processes in your mind. You will find out that as your mind becomes concentrated and accompanied with silence, it becomes easier to experience your inner awareness. With awareness, your intuition power increases. By regularly meditating, you can have an awareness of who you are and what your purpose in life is. Keep looking inside yourself, and your awareness will increase. The

_____

5   Breese, Christian D.D., Ph.D., "Pranayama & The Art of Breathing" University of Metaphysical Sciences, 2005

answer will come from within, through inner self. Everyone has an intuitive power. Meditation helps to improve the intuition in everyone who practices it and will bring you on a spiritual path. Spirituality gives you high esteem. With high esteem, you can achieve anything you want in life. There is a saying that one sees true beauty through the soul.

With meditation, you will have inner peace. It is amazing how it can lead and guide you. You have the power to accomplish anything that you want. Everything is possible, and it becomes easier to accomplish with little effort. Just as the babies start walking, the butterfly breaks from the cocoon when it's ready to start flying. If the cocoon of the butterfly is broken with effort, a butterfly will come out with crippled wings and will not be able to fly. There is a beautiful testimonial by "Deborah Saliby" on the Web regarding the cocoon of the butterfly.

Meditation relaxes the body, calms the mind, and minimizes tension. The notion of meditation helps to alleviate the thoughts in the mind. Happiness increases daily along the way. Tolerance, love, understanding, inner power, and fearlessness increase too. The concentration ability increases and the mind becomes stronger and under control. The ability to enjoy the present moment increases. One becomes humble and takes responsibility of oneself without blaming others. You become calm and a source of peace and tranquility; you start attracting people to you, as the energy you give out is high. You are no longer interested in petty gossip or wanting to know what is happening in their lives. You only forgive and love everybody and start to appreciate the small gifts that come along the way. You no longer feel disappointed with things that don't work out as you had planned, as your higher self knows best and complies passively. The materialistic aspects of life no longer drive you.

Eventually you may find that you become more mindful and more aware of everyday aspects of your life. Awareness increases. Meditation has beneficial effects on physical health. When you are meditating, your breathing becomes normal and you become more relaxed. When a body is relaxed, it breathes normally. After meditation, I get inspired to write, which puts me into a very positive mood. I continue writing for hours.

Tip No. 10
Meditation

Listen to the music and imagine you are like a feather. You are flowing, the thoughts come, and the feather does not engage with the thoughts. In other words, the thoughts come. And when the mind does not get engage with it, you just flow by it. The mind will stay free from thoughts. Daily practice of this can eliminate thoughts. You will feel naturally peaceful.

By taking long walks in nature, try to hear the sounds of birds or a water stream, or just smell the freshness of air in nature; you will feel connected with nature. Just enjoy the quiet of nature for a few hours and breathe in the new air. Simply enjoy the beauty of nature. It will take time for your mind to adjust to this silence and not listen to the jumbled noise going on in the brain of a person with a stressful life. Let go of the emotions and thoughts and try to perceive any situation in a positive manner. Doing this a few times a week will help you while meditating.

I will share another way to develop the power of concentration from the "WEL-Systems Institute".

Just allow yourself to sit back and relax in a comfortable position. And just begin to pay attention to your breathing … to the sound of your own breath … moving in and out of your body. As you breathe, just allow your breath to begin to move deeper into your body, breathing in and breathing out. Let it be easy and effortless.

And as you continue to breathe deeply into the body, imagine that your attention is a tiny, white feather, floating just above the top of your head. And then if you will imagine that as the feather sits easily above your head, the Crown chakra located directly at the top of your head begins to open ever so gently and the core of the spine begins to expand and that tiny, little white feather easily and effortlessly, ever so gently, begins to drift down all by itself right down the core of the spine, floating from side to side, like feathers do, effortless, falling easily and comfortably all the way down, right down at the base of your spine, resting ever so softly at the base of your spine. And continuing to breathe, deeply, into the base of your spine keeping your attention focused on the white feather at the base of your spine, allowing your breath to go deep into the body, all the way down to the base of the spine, and just keep breathing, as you begin to feel your body open completely ... expanding ... creating a vast, empty space inside you.[6]

When there is an empty space inside you, the energy can move freely.

Tip No. 11

Awareness

By practicing meditation regularly, we become more aware in life. By having awareness, one becomes aware of one's own mental activity. One knows the totality of one's thoughts, feelings, impressions, and expressions. To be aware, we must stop and pay attention. We need to stop and objectively watch ourselves in action. At

---

6   The *White Feather Process* is reproduced with the permission of the author and copyright holder, Louise LeBrun, founder of the WEL-Systems Institute. WEL-Systems is a registered trademark of Louise LeBrun. An audio version of this process is available on the CD set *Guided Reflections: Awakening the Body*, 2009, which is available from the WEL-Systems Institute.

the same time, keep away from low energy that is fear, anger, jealousy, gossiping, guilt, pride, ego, etc. Let go of the past, do not anticipate the future, and live in the present moment. By being nonjudgmental and by showing kindness and benevolence, you will experience high energy. You will experience your true nature, which gives you the notion of inspiration that can put you in the mode of creativity. Visualization and dreams can turn into reality.

Tip No. 12
Judging

Try saying to yourself that you will not judge anything or anybody today. To put things into perspective, soul and judging do not go together. By being on a spiritual path, judging cannot take place. In fact, by judging you hinder the spiritual path. Judging is negative. After judging someone, one does not feel good about oneself and is allowing disharmony, pain, and anger to enter one's life. This will not allow you to see things clearly.

We human beings are all one big diamond. For each facet in the diamond represents each one of us.

Let's say this big diamond is put on the earth. The facets of the diamond are facing in different directions. I am going to talk about two facets of diamond which are two people facing in opposite directions. One facet is facing the water and mountains and the other facet is facing slums and traffic. These two people perceive the world very differently because of their environment. When these two people meet, they are very different and have different views in life, but still they both can be right. So in other words, it's not good to judge somebody's behavior by saying uncomplimentary things or belittling them, because that's the only way that person knows how to behave due to his environment.

Tip No. 13
Nutrition

My doctors gave me a prescription for tamoxifen to control the estrogen level; my case of breast cancer was related to estrogen level. After my doctors told me of the side effects of tamoxifen, I decided not to take it and to use an alternate method. In the beginning, I became a vegetarian. I started eating an anti-inflammatory diet of fruits and vegetables, such as broccoli, cauliflower, cabbage, brussels sprouts, apples, etc. But now I eat chicken and meat sometimes. Organic milk is also a good dietary source.

According to research, bananas, figs, and dates are good for the function of the brain. These foods help in releasing serotonin in the brain. Serotonin gives a calming effect and makes the body feel good. Once the body feels good, one can accomplish a lot. Everything is dependent on how you control your body. If you are going through crises, talking to people is temporary, as it can alleviate the emotions, but it will come back. Being in charge and doing something about it can only eliminate the problem. If you are feeling depressed and do not feel like doing anything, light yoga can really help the body, and this will give you a calming effect. It requires lots of discipline to do yoga. But at least doing half an hour of yoga every day can be beneficial.

Tip No. 14
Breathing and Energy

As an experienced NLP (neurolinguistic programming) practitioner, I understand the relationship of mind, body, and soul. Simply put, I started breathing at the conscious level, especially when I was going through cancer. When I breathe in, my stomach inflates, and when I breathe out, my stomach relaxes. It goes in toward the spine. In order to do this kind of breathing, it creates space in the body, which in turn makes the energy move freely in the body. Most of the energy comes from oxygen and not food.

Most of the time, our lungs are not used enough with the daily tensions and stresses of life. Breathing helps the body to relax. When one is relaxed, the breathing becomes more prominent, and this helps to move the energy in the body. In order to avoid health problems, the energy has to move in the body from the brain to the stomach and back from kidneys to the brain. When you breathe at the conscious level through the stomach, the fire energy from the heart moves downward through the body to the kidneys, and the cool energy from the kidneys moves upward at the back of your spine to the brain. It relaxes the brain with the cool energy and completes the cycle.

The flow has to be smooth. The disturbance in the energy takes place when one has worries so stress and tension build up. This disturbs the normal breathing and can obstruct the flow of energy. When something obstructs the flow of energy or there is any kind of blockage, it can create stagnant energy. Any stagnant energy in the body creates different kinds of disease. The human body has a full pharmacy in it. So when one feels good about oneself, the body will go and extract the necessary chemical to help the situation. I mentioned this regarding how the brain releases serotonin when one is feeling good about oneself and laughter increases the production of the body's own painkillers.

By breathing through the stomach, the energy moves. It removes fear and depression and relaxes you. At times, one fears the future: what's going to happen, what kind of life you are going to lead, whether you will be alone or have a partner, if you will have enough money or good health to survive, etc. Fear of thinking about the future can be a waste of energy. Worrying is low energy. When you have low energy, it takes you into the past or the future. With high energy, you live more in the present.

For example, sometimes there is a moment in your life when somebody compliments you and you really feel good about yourself. It uplifts your spirits. That's a present moment, and you can accomplish anything you want. When you are in the present, you are not carrying any baggage from the past or the future. Breathing at the conscious level can also help when you are going to speak in front of an audience. If you are to give a speech or a seminar in front of a big audience, a few minutes before your time, do your breathing through your stomach. This will move your energy and will help you deliver your speech. You will not be nervous, and the speech will flow smoothly.

At times, you are late for your work or your appointment and you get the red traffic light; you panic and feel frustrated. The cells in your body are all confused and do not know what is happening. These confused cells are not good for your body. This can bring different kinds of disease to your body. The best thing to do is breathe, and automatically you will feel calm and relaxed. Even when somebody tells you to relax, still your body is all jammed with different emotions you cannot control. So when you breathe, it creates space, and automatically the energy moves and the cells in your body are feeling good. This will create a calming effect.

According to a recent survey undertaken by MIND, among people suffering from depression, many felt much better after eating a banana.[7] This is because bananas contain tryptophan, a type of protein that the body converts into serotonin, which makes you relax, improves your mood, and generally makes you feel happier.

Miracle and Focus

Life is a miracle. To be awake every morning is a miracle. A miracle is an amazing or wonderful thing or event. It can offer things to you in a miraculous way, if you know how to accept it. When you are focused, you feel good about yourself. In order to stay focused, you have to live in the present, and you will be able to accept

---

7   This topic (health benefits of bananas) is from a medical forum at snopes.com.

the great things that nature has to offer you. You will be more in tune with the notion of acceptance. When you are feeling good, it helps your mood and changes your disposition. You somehow give out a high energy to your surroundings. It's not very wise to be opinionated, which gives out the low energy. Life is a struggle and a challenge.

When you live in the present, you focus and carry out day-to-day requirements in an orderly manner. By living in the present, you give out the high energy. With the high energy, you can accomplish anything.

Tip No. 15
Attitude

"Be humble, for you are made of earth.

Be noble, for you are made of stars."

(Serbian Proverb)

With good attitude, high self-esteem kicks in and you can achieve anything easily.

Attitude

"Your living is determined not so much by what
life brings to you as by the attitude you bring to
life; not so much by what happens to you as by
the way your mind looks at what happens."

Khalil Gibran

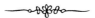

Tip No. 16
Ayurveda

The information below is from a study at the School of
Ayurveda and Panchakarma, Kannur District, Kerala
State, South India. I am an Ayurvedic master and did a
diploma course at the mentioned school.

Ayurveda is the natural healing system of India dating
back to BC 3000.

The Sanskrit term *Ayurveda* is composed of two
words: *ayu* and *veda*. Ayu means life, and veda means
knowledge or science. So the two words combine to give
the meaning "the science of life," "the knowledge about
life," or "a sensible way of living."

Unique Features of Ayurveda

1. Treat the root cause of the disease.

2. Medicines are free from toxicity.

3. The same treatments can be done for the diseased as well as the healthy.

4. The medicines are less expensive.

5. Emphasis on preventive medicine.

6. Ayurveda is near to nature.

7. Yoga and Ayurveda.

8. Simple methods of diagnosis.

9. Detoxification treatments.

The Aim of Ayurveda

1. Relief of the misery of suffering people.

2. Preservation of the health of healthy people.

When to Eat

One should only eat when one is hungry. In other words, eat when the fire (*agni*) is burning. Then only will the food be cooked and digested. If there is no agni, the food will not be cooked and will not digest, so the food will turn into toxins. In other words, the food will be sitting in your stomach and turn into toxins, the same as if you had left food out on the counter for a few days. It is also important what time of the day you eat. If you eat late at night, you will feel lethargic the next day, because the food was not cooked properly. This is due to the lack of agni (fire) as the body slows down toward the evening. Proper digestion cannot take place, as the body is working to burn off toxins and continues to digest the food from the day.

Ayurveda seems to connect our mind and body with the environment, nature's clock. Living in harmony with nature is the Ayurvedic style of living, which promotes health and happiness in our body. Wake up early with the sunrise, and go to sleep by 10:00 p.m. Waking up early helps to prevent a depressed mood, and at that time the communication between heart and mind is clearer.

One way to know if your body has toxins is when the stool sinks. There are no toxins when the stool floats.

In Ayurveda, three *doshas* are the components that carry over the functions of the body. The three doshas are Vata, Pitha, and Kapha. Which dosha you are can be determined by answering a questionnaire and by taking the pulse. Contact the author.

Six tastes of food are connected with the three doshas. The six tastes, according to Ayurveda, are sweet, sour, salty, bitter, pungent, and astringent.

The six tastes of food taken in every meal balance the doshas.

	Most Balancing	**Most Aggravating**
Vata	Sweet, sour, salty	Bitter, pungent, astringent
Pitha	Sweet, bitter, astringent	Sour, salty, pungent
Kapha	Pungent, bitter, astringent	Sweet, sour, salty

Sweet has a soothing effect to the body: fruit, grains, pasta, rice, honey, dairy, etc.

Sour foods are citrus fruits, yogurt, fermented foods, alcohol, etc.

Salt improves taste: natural salts, soy sauce, etc.

Bitter helps in detoxifying the body: green leafy vegetables, broccoli, beets, celery, etc.

Pungent enhances sweating and clears sinuses: chili peppers, garlic, onions, cayenne, black pepper, cloves, etc.

Astringent tightens tissues: lentils, green apples, pomegranates, etc.

The three doshas are divided into three sections in the body.

Kapha dosha: chest, throat, head, joints, stomach, small intestine, plasma, muscles, bone marrow, sperm or ovum, nose, and tongue. For example, a cold is a Kapha disease that occurs when the Kapha is aggravated.

Pitha dosha: navel, stomach, small intestine, sweat, blood, eyes, and skin. Any issues with stomach, blood, etc. are due to Pitha being aggravated.

Vata dosha: the lower part of the body, which includes the large intestine, waist, thighs, bones, ears, and skin. Joint problems, arthritis, etc. are due to Vata being aggravated.

Final Thoughts: Tamed the Lion

Upon reflection, I feel good, because after nine years, I am still healthy. And I am pleased to report that I still do all the good things today that I did during my journey. Living a spiritual life and using the techniques that I discussed in this book helped me give my body the ammunition it needed to fight the cancer and ultimately "silence the roar of lions."

As the reader of my book, I hope that you will take these tips and use them to help yourself. I wish you a speedy recovery and a healthy life.

Poem about 3 months at the Ayurveda School in India

Arriving first time in India at the Calicutt airport,

Intrigued to see only Indians, same colour,
with smiling faces ready to help.

Kannur in Kerala was the place where
Ayurvedic school was in the centre town,

Where hustle and bustle of cars, buses and rickshas,

Never heard so much honking ever before.

Students from different countries i.e. Germany,
France, Ireland, etc. With different, backgrounds
and different age groups all in one class.

From climbing 4 flights of stairs with heavy bag on
the shoulder to learn Ayurveda, Where breaks were
not given on time and was looked at it positively,

How utterly wonderful all this is.

Lunch times were great, buying
mangoes, guavas, all so sweet,

Was eaten quickly and greedily,

Honking of cars were immuned to the
ears and I felt part of the crowd.

Dogs and cats were walking and crossing
roads lazily and also felt part of the crowd,

Not being kicked around as long as
they did not harm others.

Living in front of the Arabian Sea which was not
a tourist area, seeing locals peeing on the rocks, in
a natural air freshner, a real connection with the
nature and no artificial air freshner was required.

Trip to the school with other students in the school van
was exciting with Indian filmy songs playing very loud
in the morning, no excuse to be sleepy in the class.

Any excuse to have a party with
dancing, lots of food and fun.

Parties always ended at midnight, after taking
a dip in the Arabian Sea with the joyous
crowd, talking at the highest pitch.

Even the snakes got frightened
and hid under the rocks,

So were the Lovely Days in India.

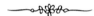

About the Author

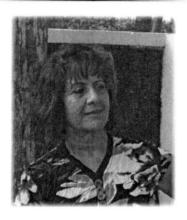

Nazmina Ladhani is following an online degree course in metaphysics with the University of Metaphysical Sciences in California. She is an Ayurvedic master and did a diploma course at School of Ayurveda and Panchakarma, Kannur District, Kerala State, South India. She is a qualified yoga teacher and followed the course at Chopra University in Carlsbad, California. Nazmina is an NLP (neuro-linguistic programming) practitioner and did a course at Well Systems Institute in Ottawa. She worked several years for the Federal Government of Canada and was born in Kampala, Uganda, East Africa.

CPSIA information can be obtained at www.ICGtesting.com
Printed in the USA
LVOW080349080513

332721LV00001B/1/P